Vibrant Living

Tasty and Nourishing Recipes for Those Over 50 Managing Diabetes

Dr. Brandon .C

Table of content

INTRODUCTION

As we journey through life, our bodies undergo numerous changes, and for many individuals, the milestone of turning 50 marks a significant transition. It's a time when we reflect on our health, our habits, and our future. For those managing diabetes, this stage can bring about unique challenges and opportunities for proactive health management.

Diabetic Diet After 50 is more than just a cookbook; it's a guide crafted with care and consideration for those navigating the complexities of diabetes in their golden years. In this introduction, we'll explore the importance of understanding diabetes after 50, the pivotal role diet plays in managing this condition, the key components of a diabetic-friendly diet, and practical tips for creating meals that are both simple and nourishing.

Understanding Diabetes After 50

Diabetes is a chronic condition characterized by high blood sugar levels, often resulting from the body's inability to produce or effectively use insulin. While diabetes can develop at any age, the risk increases with age, and many individuals find themselves facing this diagnosis later in life.

After 50, the body's metabolism may slow down, making it more challenging to regulate blood sugar levels. Additionally, other age-related factors such as decreased physical activity, changes in muscle mass, and potential complications from other health conditions can further complicate diabetes management.

Understanding the unique aspects of diabetes after 50 is crucial for effectively managing the condition and maintaining overall health and well-being. It involves recognizing the importance of lifestyle factors, including diet, exercise, stress management, and regular medical care, in controlling blood sugar levels and reducing the risk of complications.

Importance of Diet in Managing Diabetes

Among the various factors influencing diabetes management, diet plays a central role. The foods we eat directly impact our blood sugar levels, insulin sensitivity, and overall health. For individuals over 50 living with diabetes, adopting a healthy eating plan is essential for stabilizing blood sugar levels, managing weight, reducing the risk of cardiovascular complications, and promoting overall well-being.

A diabetic-friendly diet focuses on balancing carbohydrates, proteins, and fats while emphasizing whole, nutrient-dense foods. It prioritizes complex carbohydrates with a low glycemic index, lean proteins, healthy fats, and an abundance of fruits and vegetables. By choosing foods that support stable blood sugar levels and provide essential nutrients, individuals can better manage their diabetes and enjoy improved energy levels, mood, and overall health.

Key Components of a Diabetic-Friendly Diet

Crafting a diabetic-friendly diet after 50 involves paying attention to several key components:

1. **Carbohydrates:** Choosing carbohydrates that are high in fiber and low in sugar can help prevent spikes in blood sugar levels. Whole grains, legumes, fruits, and vegetables are excellent choices.

2. **Proteins:** Including lean sources of protein such as poultry, fish, tofu, and legumes can help stabilize blood sugar levels and promote satiety.

3. **Fats:** Opting for healthy fats from sources like avocados, nuts, seeds, and olive oil can support heart health and improve insulin sensitivity.

4. **Portion Control:** Managing portion sizes is essential for controlling calorie intake and preventing blood sugar fluctuations.

5. **Hydration:** Staying hydrated with water and avoiding sugary beverages is important for overall health and blood sugar management.

6. **Consistency:** Establishing regular meal times and spacing meals evenly throughout the day can help stabilize blood sugar levels and prevent overeating.

Tips for Creating Simple and Easy Diabetic Meals

Creating simple and easy diabetic meals doesn't have to be complicated. With a few practical tips and a bit of creativity, you can enjoy delicious and nutritious meals that support your health and well-being:

Plan Ahead: Take the time to plan your meals and snacks for the week, making sure to include a balance of carbohydrates, proteins, and fats.

Batch Cooking: Prepare large batches of staple foods such as grains, proteins, and vegetables ahead of time, so you have ingredients ready to assemble into meals throughout the week.

Choose Convenience Foods Wisely: Opt for convenience foods that are minimally processed and low in added sugars, salt, and unhealthy fats.

Experiment with Flavors:

Don't be afraid to experiment with herbs, spices, and healthy condiments to add flavor to your meals without adding extra sugar or salt.

1. **Stay Mindful of Portions:** Use smaller plates and utensils to help control portion sizes and prevent overeating.

2. **Listen to Your Body:** Pay attention to how different foods affect your blood sugar levels and adjust your diet accordingly. Be sure to consult with a healthcare professional or registered dietitian for personalized guidance.

In "Simple and Easy Diabetic Diet After 50," we've curated a collection of 30 delicious recipes designed specifically with the needs and preferences of individuals over 50 in mind. From hearty breakfasts to satisfying entrees and indulgent desserts, these recipes are not only simple to prepare but also packed with flavor and nutrition.

Whether you're newly diagnosed with diabetes or have been managing the condition for years, this cookbook serves as a valuable resource for embracing a healthier lifestyle and taking control of your health after 50.

By incorporating these recipes into your meal rotation and making mindful choices every day, you can nourish your body, stabilize your blood sugar levels, and enjoy a vibrant and fulfilling life.

So, let's embark on this journey together, celebrating the joy of nourishing our bodies, embracing healthy habits, and savoring the simple pleasures of delicious food. Here's to your health, happiness, and longevity!

1

Breakfast Ideas

Breakfast is often hailed as the most important meal of the day, and for good reason. It kick-starts your metabolism, provides you with energy to start your day, and can set the tone for healthy eating habits throughout the day. For individuals over 50 managing diabetes, a balanced and nutritious breakfast is essential for stabilizing blood sugar levels and supporting overall health.

In this chapter, we've compiled a selection of five delicious breakfast ideas that are not only simple to prepare but also packed with flavor and nutrition. From hearty parfaits to savory omelettes and satisfying oatmeal, these recipes are designed to help you start your day off right, providing you with the energy and nourishment you need to thrive. So, grab your apron and let's dive into a world of delicious and diabetes-friendly breakfast options!

Berry and Greek Yogurt Parfait

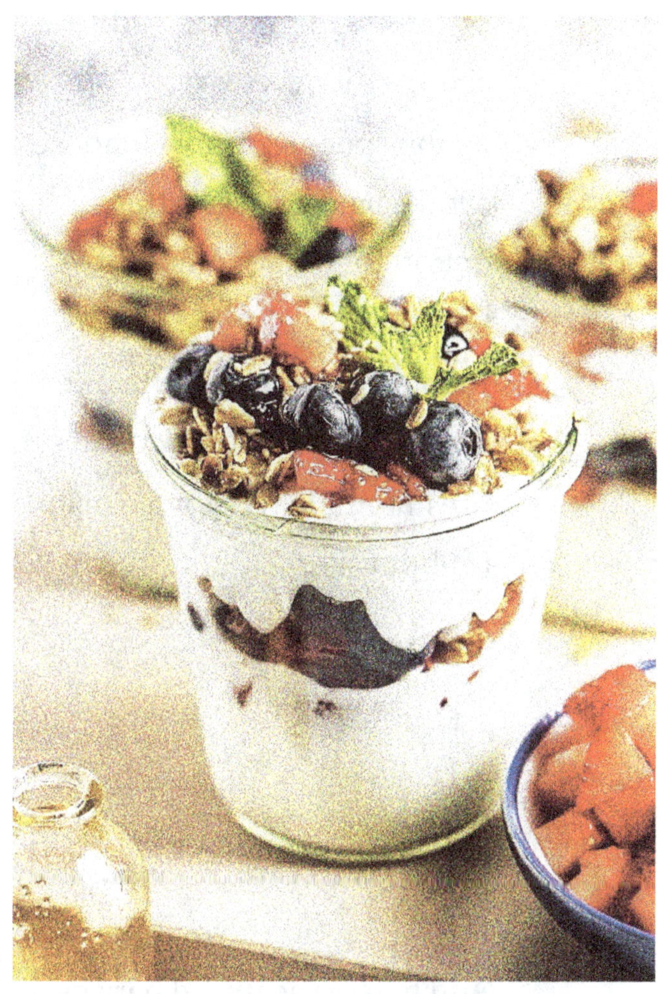

Time of Preparation: 10 minutes
Serving Unit: 1 parfait

Ingredients

* 1/2 cup Greek yogurt (plain, unsweetened)
* 1/4 cup mixed berries (such as strawberries, blueberries, and raspberries), washed and chopped if necessary
* 2 tablespoons granola (choose a low-sugar or sugar-free option for diabetic-friendly version)
* 1 tablespoon honey or maple syrup (optional, for sweetness)
* Fresh mint leaves for garnish (optional)

Procedure

1. In a small bowl or glass, layer half of the Greek yogurt.
2. Add half of the mixed berries on top of the yogurt layer.
3. Sprinkle half of the granola over the berries.
4. Repeat the layers with the remaining yogurt, berries, and granola.
5. Drizzle honey or maple syrup over the top layer if desired.
6. Garnish with fresh mint leaves for a pop of color and flavor.
7. Serve immediately and enjoy!

Nutritional Value (per serving)

* Calories: 200
* Protein: 12g
* Fat: 4g
* Carbohydrates: 30g
* Fiber: 4g
* Sugars: 15g

Cooking Tips

* Use plain, unsweetened Greek yogurt to control the amount of added sugar.
* Opt for fresh or frozen mixed berries, depending on availability and preference.
* Choose a granola that is low in added sugars and high in fiber for a healthier option.

- Customize your parfait by adding nuts, seeds, or a sprinkle of cinnamon for extra flavor and texture.

Health Benefits

Rich in Protein: Greek yogurt is an excellent source of protein, which helps promote satiety and regulate blood sugar levels.

Loaded with Antioxidants: Berries are packed with antioxidants, vitamins, and minerals that support overall health and may help reduce inflammation.

Good Source of Fiber: Both Greek yogurt and berries contain dietary fiber, which aids in digestion, promotes gut health, and helps control blood sugar levels.

Low Glycemic Index: This parfait has a low glycemic index, meaning it won't cause a rapid spike in blood sugar levels, making it suitable for individuals managing diabetes.

Balanced Nutrition: With a balance of protein, carbohydrates, and fats, this parfait provides a well-rounded meal to kick-start your day while keeping blood sugar levels stable.

Enjoy this Berry and Greek Yogurt Parfait as a nutritious and satisfying breakfast option that's both delicious and diabetes-friendly.

Veggie Omelette with Spinach and Mushrooms

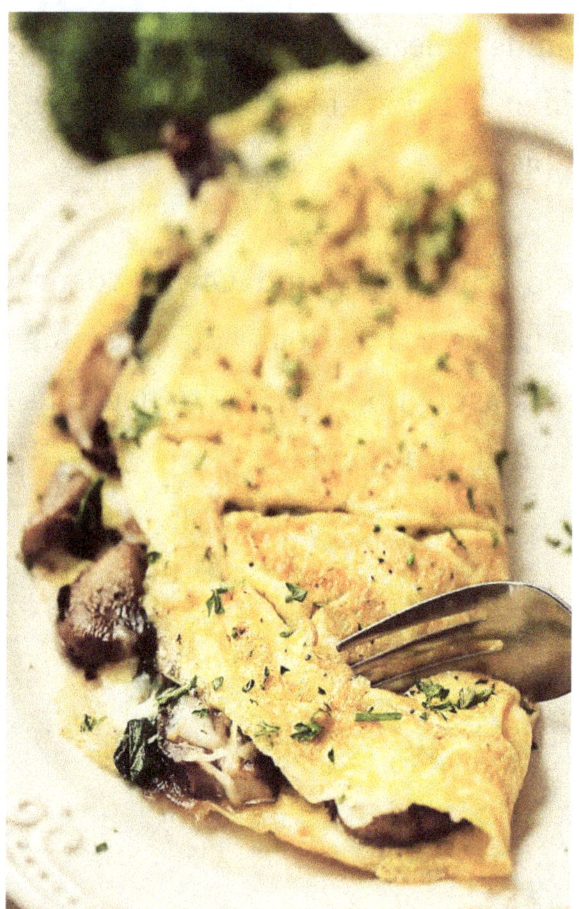

Time of Preparation: 15 minutes
Cooking Time: 10 minutes
Serving Unit: 1 omelette

Ingredients

- 2 large eggs
- 1/4 cup spinach, chopped
- 1/4 cup mushrooms, sliced
- 1/4 cup bell peppers, diced
- 1 tablespoon olive oil
- Salt and pepper to taste
- Optional: shredded cheese for topping (choose a low-fat option for healthier version)

Procedure:

1. In a bowl, beat the eggs until well combined. Season with salt and pepper to taste.
2. Heat olive oil in a non-stick skillet over medium heat.
3. Add the mushrooms and bell peppers to the skillet and sauté for 2-3 minutes until softened.
4. Add the chopped spinach to the skillet and cook for another 1-2 minutes until wilted.

5. Pour the beaten eggs over the vegetables in the skillet, spreading them out evenly.

6. Cook the omelette for 3-4 minutes, lifting the edges with a spatula and tilting the skillet to allow uncooked eggs to flow underneath.

7. Once the eggs are mostly set, sprinkle shredded cheese over one half of the omelette if using.

8. Carefully fold the omelette in half using a spatula and cook for another 1-2 minutes until the cheese is melted and the eggs are cooked through.

9. Slide the omelette onto a plate and serve hot.

Nutritional Value (per serving):

- Calories: 250
- Protein: 15g
- Fat: 18g
- Carbohydrates: 5g
- Fiber: 2g
- Sugars: 2g

Cooking Tips:

- Use a non-stick skillet to prevent the omelette from sticking.
- Customize the omelette with your favorite vegetables such as tomatoes, onions, or broccoli.
- Be mindful of the amount of cheese used to control calories and fat intake.
- Serve with a side of whole grain toast or fresh fruit for a complete meal.

Health Benefits:

High in Protein: Eggs are an excellent source of high-quality protein, which helps build and repair tissues in the body.

Packed with Vegetables: This omelette is loaded with nutrient-rich vegetables like spinach, mushrooms, and bell peppers, providing essential vitamins, minerals, and antioxidants.

Good Source of Fiber: Vegetables like spinach and mushrooms contribute dietary fiber, which supports digestion and promotes satiety.

Heart-Healthy Fats: Olive oil used for cooking provides heart-healthy monounsaturated fats, which may help reduce the risk of cardiovascular disease.

Low in Carbohydrates: With minimal carbohydrates, this veggie omelette is suitable for individuals following a low-carb or diabetic-friendly diet.

Enjoy this Veggie Omelette with Spinach and Mushrooms as a nutritious and satisfying breakfast option that's both delicious and easy to prepare.

Overnight Oats with Chia Seeds and Almond Milk

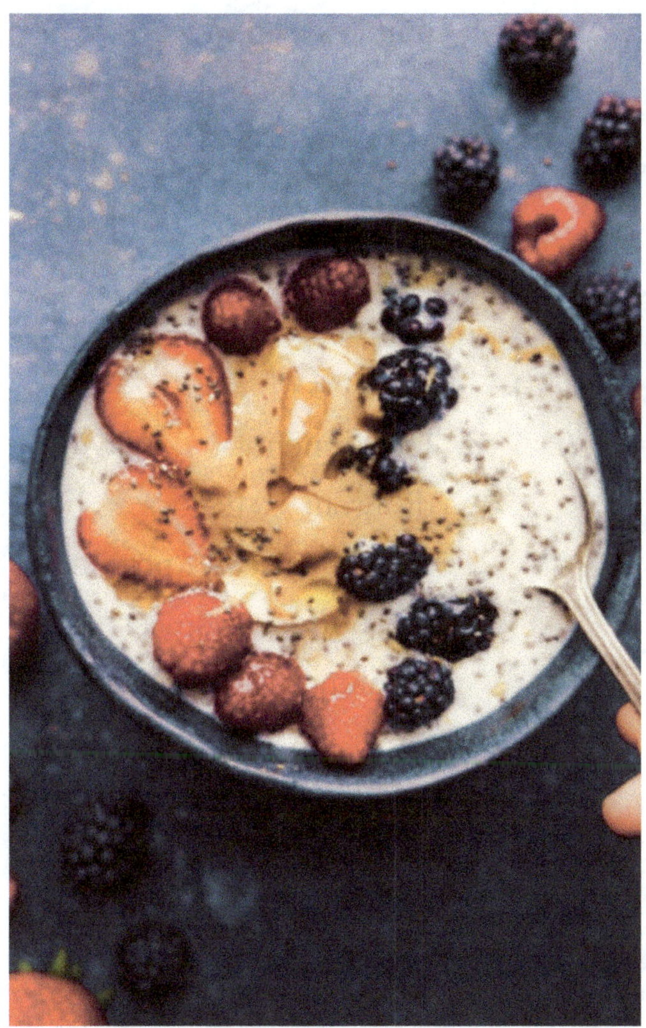

Time of Preparation: 5 minutes (plus overnight soaking)

Serving Unit: 1 bowl

Ingredients:

- 1/2 cup rolled oats (old-fashioned oats)
- 1 tablespoon chia seeds
- 1/2 cup unsweetened almond milk (or any milk of choice)
- 1/4 teaspoon vanilla extract
- 1 tablespoon honey or maple syrup (optional, for sweetness)
- Fresh fruit for topping (such as berries, sliced banana, or chopped apple)

Procedure:

1. In a bowl or jar, combine rolled oats, chia seeds, almond milk, vanilla extract, and honey or maple syrup if using. Stir until well combined.
2. Cover the bowl or jar with a lid or plastic wrap and refrigerate overnight or for at least 4 hours to allow the oats and chia seeds to soak and soften.

3. Before serving, give the overnight oats a stir and add more almond milk if desired to achieve your preferred consistency.
4. Top the overnight oats with fresh fruit of your choice.
5. Serve cold and enjoy!

Nutritional Value (per serving):

- Calories: 250
- Protein: 7g
- Fat: 8g
- Carbohydrates: 40g
- Fiber: 8g
- Sugars: 10g

Cooking Tips:

a. Customize your overnight oats with various toppings such as nuts, seeds, coconut flakes, or a sprinkle of cinnamon.
b. Adjust the sweetness according to your preference by adding more or less honey or maple syrup.
c. Use a mason jar for convenient storage and easy transportation if you're making the overnight oats ahead of time.
d. Experiment with different flavors by adding cocoa powder, nut butter, or spices like cinnamon or nutmeg.

Health Benefits:

Rich in Fiber: Both oats and chia seeds are rich in soluble fiber, which helps promote digestive health, regulate blood sugar levels, and keep you feeling full and satisfied.

Good Source of Plant-Based Protein: Chia seeds provide plant-based protein, which is essential for muscle repair and growth.

Low Glycemic Index: This breakfast has a low glycemic index, meaning it won't cause a rapid spike in blood sugar levels, making it suitable for individuals managing diabetes.

Heart-Healthy Fats: Chia seeds contain omega-3 fatty acids, which are beneficial for heart health and may help reduce inflammation.

Convenient and Portable: Overnight oats are a convenient breakfast option that can be prepared ahead of time and enjoyed on the go, making them perfect for busy mornings.

Start your day off right with these delicious and nutritious Overnight Oats with Chia Seeds and Almond Milk, packed with fiber, protein, and essential nutrients.

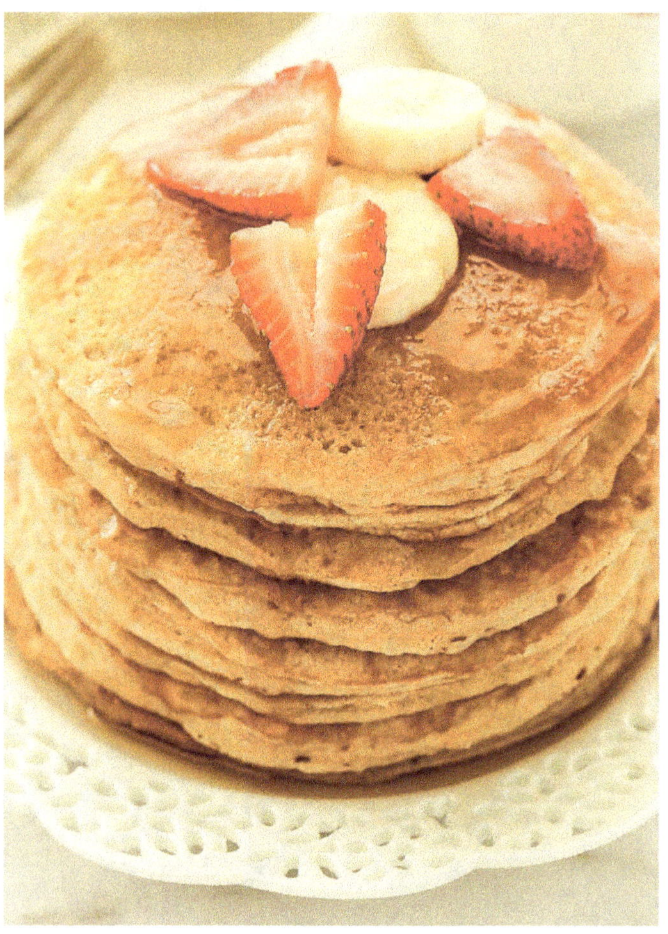

Time of Preparation: 20 minutes
Cooking Time: 10 minutes
Serving Unit: 2 pancakes

Ingredients:

- 1 cup whole wheat flour
- 1 tablespoon baking powder
- 1 tablespoon honey or maple syrup
- 1 cup unsweetened almond milk (or any milk of choice)
- 1 large egg
- 1 tablespoon olive oil or melted butter
- 1 teaspoon vanilla extract
- Sugar-free pancake syrup for serving

Procedure:

1. In a large bowl, whisk together whole wheat flour and baking powder.
2. In a separate bowl, beat the egg and add almond milk, honey or maple syrup, olive oil or melted butter, and vanilla extract. Whisk until well combined.
3. Pour the wet ingredients into the dry ingredients and stir

until just combined. Be careful not to overmix; a few lumps are okay.

4. Heat a non-stick skillet or griddle over medium heat and lightly grease with cooking spray or oil.
5. Pour about 1/4 cup of the pancake batter onto the skillet for each pancake.
6. Cook until bubbles form on the surface of the pancakes and the edges look set, about 2-3 minutes.
7. Flip the pancakes and cook for an additional 1-2 minutes until golden brown and cooked through.
8. Remove the pancakes from the skillet and keep warm while you cook the remaining batter.
9. Serve the whole wheat pancakes warm with sugar-free pancake syrup or your favorite topping.

Nutritional Value (per serving, Two pancakes)

- Calories: 250
- Protein: 8g
- Fat: 6g
- Carbohydrates: 40g
- Fiber: 6g
- Sugars: 4g

Cooking Tips:

1. Be sure not to overmix the batter, as this can result in tough pancakes. It's okay if there are a few lumps in the batter.
2. Use a non-stick skillet or griddle to prevent the pancakes from sticking.
3. Adjust the consistency of the batter by adding more milk if it's too thick or more flour if it's too thin.
4. Keep the pancakes warm in a preheated oven while you cook the remaining batches.

Health Benefits:

Whole Grains: Whole wheat flour used in these pancakes provides fiber, vitamins, minerals, and antioxidants that are beneficial for heart health and digestion.

Low Glycemic Index: Whole wheat pancakes have a lower glycemic index compared to pancakes made with refined flour, meaning they have a slower impact on blood sugar levels.

Protein-Rich: Eggs in the pancake batter add protein, which helps promote satiety and supports muscle repair and growth.

Heart-Healthy Fats: Olive oil or melted butter used in the batter provides monounsaturated fats, which are beneficial for heart health.

Controlled Sugar Intake: Using sugar-free pancake syrup reduces the added sugar content of the dish, making it suitable for individuals managing diabetes or watching their sugar intake.

Indulge in these Whole Wheat Pancakes with Sugar-Free Syrup for a wholesome and satisfying breakfast option that's both delicious and nutritious.

Avocado Toast with Poached Egg

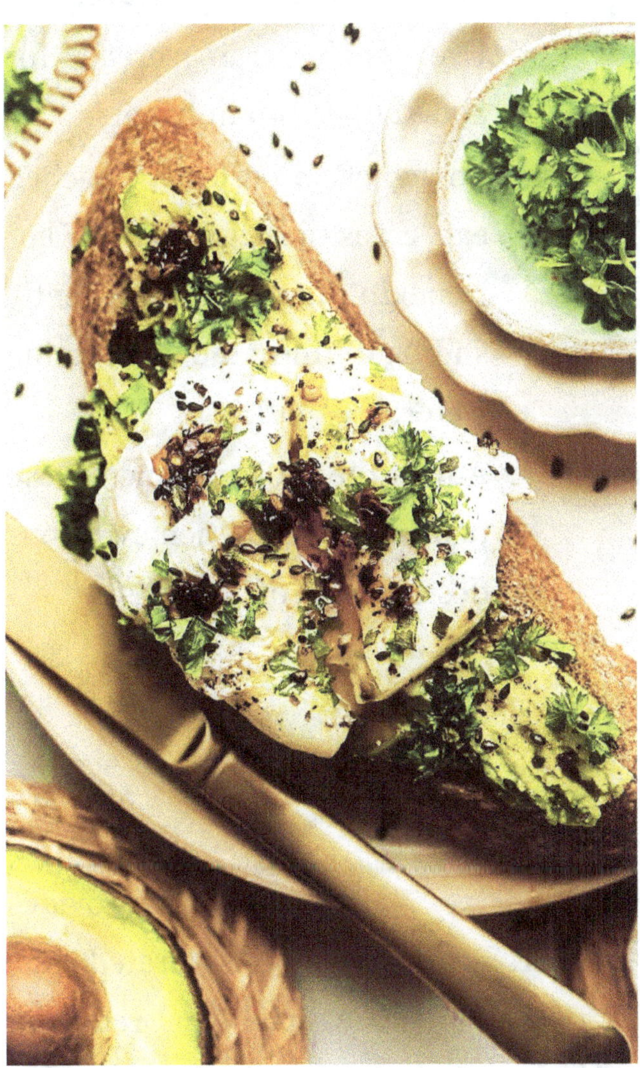

Time of Preparation: 10 minutes
Cooking Time: 5 minutes
Serving Unit: 1 serving

Ingredients:

- 1 slice whole grain bread, toasted
- 1/2 ripe avocado, mashed
- 1 large egg
- Salt and pepper to taste
- Red pepper flakes for garnish (optional)
- Fresh cilantro or parsley for garnish (optional)

Procedure:

1. Toast the slice of whole grain bread until golden brown and crispy.
2. While the bread is toasting, bring a small pot of water to a simmer over medium heat.
3. Crack the egg into a small bowl or ramekin.
4. Once the water is simmering, gently slide the egg into the pot and cook for 3-4 minutes for a soft poached egg or 5-6 minutes for a firmer poached egg.

5. While the egg is poaching, spread the mashed avocado evenly on the toasted bread.

6. Using a slotted spoon, carefully remove the poached egg from the water and drain off any excess water.

7. Place the poached egg on top of the mashed avocado.

8. Season the poached egg with salt, pepper, and red pepper flakes if desired.

9. Garnish with fresh cilantro or parsley if using.

10. Serve the avocado toast with poached egg immediately while warm.

Nutritional Value (per serving):

- Calories: 250
- Protein: 12g
- Fat: 15g
- Carbohydrates: 20g
- Fiber: 6g
- Sugars: 2g

Cooking Tips:

- Choose ripe avocados for optimal flavor and texture.
- Use whole grain bread for added fiber and nutrients.
- To achieve a perfectly poached egg, crack the egg into a bowl or ramekin first before gently sliding it into the simmering water.
- Adjust the cooking time for the poached egg to achieve your desired level of doneness.

Health Benefits:

Healthy Fats: Avocado provides heart-healthy monounsaturated fats, which are beneficial for reducing inflammation and improving cholesterol levels.

Protein: Eggs are an excellent source of high-quality protein, which helps keep you feeling full and satisfied.

Fiber: Whole grain bread and avocado are both rich in fiber, which supports digestive health and helps regulate blood sugar levels.

Vitamins and Minerals: Avocado is a good source of vitamins E, K, and B6, as well as folate and potassium, while eggs provide essential nutrients such as vitamin D, vitamin B12, and selenium.

Satiety: The combination of protein, healthy fats, and fiber in this dish makes it a satisfying breakfast option that can help curb cravings and prevent overeating later in the day.

Enjoy this Avocado Toast with Poached Egg as a delicious and nutritious breakfast or brunch option that's both simple to prepare and packed with flavor and wholesome ingredients.

2

Lunch Recipe

Lunch is an important meal that provides our bodies with the fuel they need to function properly and keeps us going for the rest of the day. Within the scope of "Chapter 2: Lunch Recipes," we delve into a compilation of scrumptious and wholesome dishes that are intended to titillate your taste buds while simultaneously supplying you with the energy and nourishment you require to power through the afternoon.

These lunch recipes have been carefully crafted to offer a balance of flavors, textures, and nutrients. For example, they include hearty wraps, vibrant salads, and comforting soups. You will find both inspiration and practicality in this varied collection of recipes, whether you are using them to prepare a lunch to take with you on the go or to enjoy a leisurely midday meal at home.

We invite you to join us as we delve into the art of preparing scrumptious and wholesome lunches that are not only easy to prepare but also fulfilling to consume and are crafted to promote your health and well-being. A celebration of good food, good health, and the joy of nourishing your body with wholesome ingredients and vibrant flavors, this chapter is a celebration from the very beginning to the very end.

Grilled Chicken Salad with Balsamic Vinaigrette

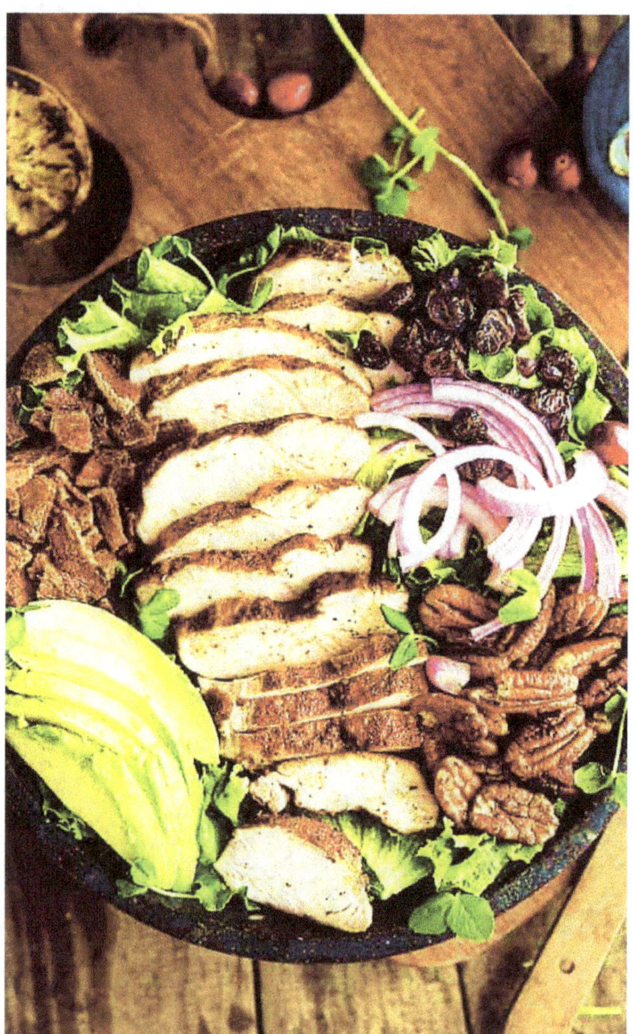

Time of Preparation: 20 minutes
Cooking Time: 15 minutes
Serving Unit: 1 salad

Ingredients:

- 4 oz grilled chicken breast, sliced
- 2 cups mixed salad greens (such as lettuce, spinach, and arugula)
- 1/2 cup cherry tomatoes, halved
- 1/4 cup cucumber, sliced
- 1/4 cup red onion, thinly sliced
- 1/4 cup carrots, shredded
- 2 tablespoons balsamic vinaigrette dressing (store-bought or homemade)
- Salt and pepper to taste
- Optional: crumbled feta cheese or sliced avocado for topping

Procedure:

1. Season the chicken breast with salt and pepper, then grill until cooked through, about 6-8 minutes per side. Allow the chicken to rest for

a few minutes before slicing it thinly.

2. In a large bowl, combine the mixed salad greens, cherry tomatoes, cucumber, red onion, and shredded carrots.
3. Add the sliced grilled chicken to the salad.
4. Drizzle the balsamic vinaigrette dressing over the salad and toss gently to coat.
5. Divide the salad into serving bowls and top with crumbled feta cheese or sliced avocado if desired.
6. Serve immediately and enjoy!

Nutritional Value (per serving):

- Calories: 300
- Protein: 25g
- Fat: 12g
- Carbohydrates: 20g
- Fiber: 5g
- Sugars: 10g

Cooking Tips:

1. Use leftover grilled chicken or pre-cooked chicken for a quicker preparation time.
2. Customize the salad with your favorite vegetables or toppings such as bell peppers, olives, or nuts.
3. Make your own balsamic vinaigrette dressing by whisking together balsamic vinegar, olive oil, Dijon mustard, honey, salt, and pepper.
4. To keep the salad fresh and crisp, dress it just before serving.

Health Benefits:

Lean Protein: Grilled chicken breast is a lean source of protein, which helps build and repair tissues, support muscle growth, and keep you feeling full and satisfied.

Nutrient-Dense Vegetables: The salad is packed with nutrient-rich vegetables like cherry tomatoes, cucumber, red onion, and carrots, providing essential vitamins, minerals, and antioxidants.

Low-Calorie Dressing: Balsamic vinaigrette dressing adds flavor to the salad without significantly increasing the calorie count. It's lower in fat and calories compared to creamy dressings.

High Fiber: The combination of vegetables and greens in the salad provides dietary fiber, which supports digestion, regulates blood sugar levels, and promotes satiety.

Heart-Healthy Fats: Adding sliced avocado or crumbled feta cheese to the salad provides healthy fats, including monounsaturated fats and omega-3 fatty acids, which are beneficial for heart health.

Indulge in this Grilled Chicken Salad with Balsamic Vinaigrette for a light yet satisfying lunch option that's bursting with flavor and nutrition.

Quinoa and Black Bean Stuffed Bell Peppers

- 1/2 cup quinoa, rinsed
- 1 cup water or vegetable broth
- 1 can (15 oz) black beans, drained and rinsed
- 1 cup corn kernels (fresh, canned, or frozen)
- 1/2 cup bell peppers, diced
- 1/4 cup red onion, diced
- 2 cloves garlic, minced
- 1 teaspoon ground cumin
- 1/2 teaspoon chili powder
- Salt and pepper to taste
- 2 large bell peppers, halved and seeds removed
- 1/2 cup shredded cheese (such as cheddar or Monterey Jack)
- Fresh cilantro for garnish (optional)
- Lime wedges for serving (optional)

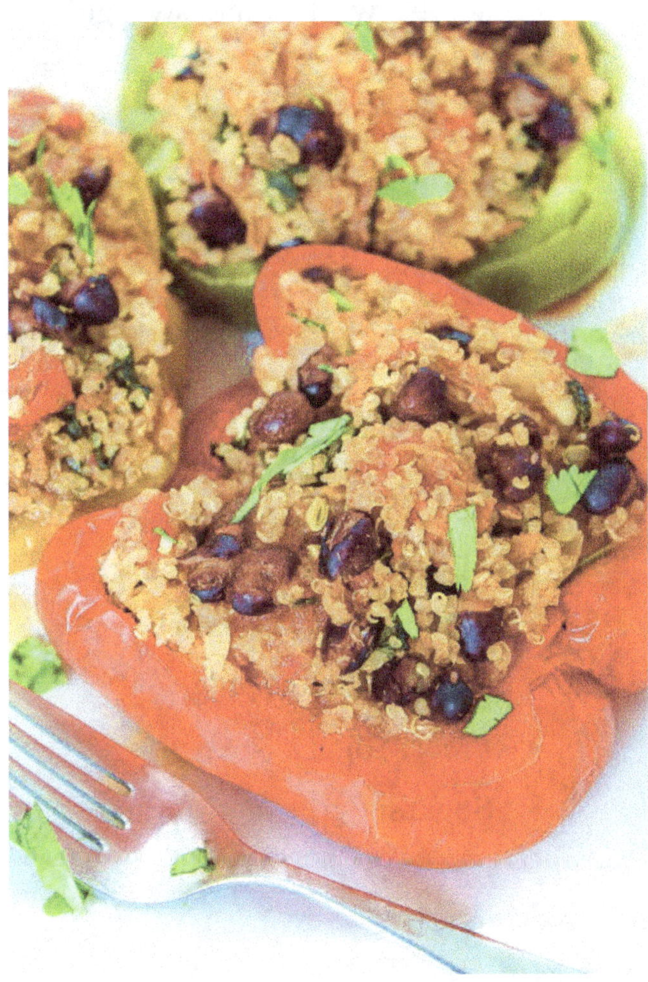

Time of Preparation: 20 minutes

Cooking Time: 30 minutes

Serving Unit: 2 stuffed bell peppers

Ingredients:

Procedure:

1. In a medium saucepan, combine quinoa and water or vegetable broth. Bring to a boil, then reduce heat to low, cover,

and simmer for 15 minutes or until quinoa is cooked and water is absorbed.

2. In a large skillet, heat olive oil over medium heat. Add diced bell peppers, red onion, and minced garlic, and sauté until softened, about 5 minutes.

3. Add cooked quinoa, black beans, corn kernels, ground cumin, chili powder, salt, and pepper to the skillet. Stir to combine and cook for another 2-3 minutes until heated through.

4. Preheat the oven to 375°F (190°C).

5. Place the halved bell peppers in a baking dish, cut side up.

6. Spoon the quinoa and black bean mixture evenly into each bell pepper half.

7. Sprinkle shredded cheese over the stuffed bell peppers.

8. Cover the baking dish with aluminum foil and bake for 20-25 minutes until the bell peppers are tender and the cheese is melted and bubbly.

9. Remove the foil and bake for an additional 5 minutes until the cheese is golden brown.

10. Garnish with fresh cilantro and serve with lime wedges if desired.

Nutritional Value (per serving, One stuffed bell pepper):

- Calories: 300
- Protein: 12g
- Fat: 8g
- Carbohydrates: 45g
- Fiber: 10g
- Sugars: 6g

Cooking Tips:

1. Use any color of bell peppers for variety and visual appeal.

2. Customize the filling by adding your favorite vegetables or spices.

3. For a vegan version, omit the cheese or use dairy-free cheese alternative.

4. Make a double batch of the quinoa and black bean filling and freeze the extra for future meals.

Health Benefits:

Plant-Based Protein: Quinoa and black beans provide plant-based protein, which is essential for muscle repair and growth.

High in Fiber: Both quinoa and black beans are rich in dietary fiber, which supports digestive health, regulates blood sugar levels, and promotes satiety.

Nutrient-Dense: This dish is packed with a variety of vegetables, including bell peppers, onions, and corn, providing essential vitamins, minerals, and antioxidants.

Low in Fat: With minimal added fat, this recipe is relatively low in calories and fat, making it suitable for individuals watching their fat intake or looking to maintain a healthy weight.

Balanced Meal: Quinoa and black beans are complex carbohydrates that provide sustained energy, while the addition of vegetables adds volume, flavor, and additional nutrients to the meal.

Savor the flavors of these Quinoa and Black Bean Stuffed Bell Peppers for a hearty and nutritious lunch option that's both satisfying and wholesome.

Turkey and Hummus Wrap with Whole Wheat Tortilla

Time of Preparation: 15 minus

Serving Unit: 1 wrap

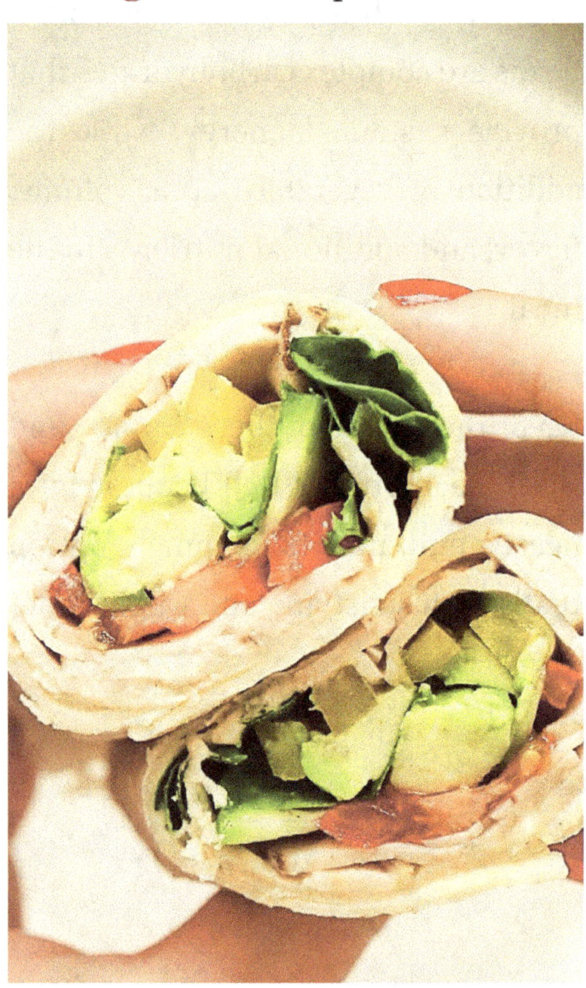

Ingredients:

- 1 whole wheat tortilla (8-inch)
- 2 tablespoons hummus (store-bought or homemade)
- 3 oz sliced turkey breast
- 1/4 cup shredded lettuce
- 1/4 cup cucumber, thinly sliced
- 1/4 cup tomato, diced
- 1 tablespoon red onion, thinly sliced
- Salt and pepper to taste
- Optional: sliced avocado or roasted red peppers for extra flavor

Procedure:

1. Spread the hummus evenly over the whole wheat tortilla, leaving a border around the edges.
2. Layer the sliced turkey breast, shredded lettuce, cucumber slices, diced tomato, and sliced red onion on top of the hummus.
3. Season with salt and pepper to taste.

4. If using, add sliced avocado or roasted red peppers for extra flavor and nutrition.
5. Roll up the tortilla tightly, tucking in the sides as you go to enclose the filling.
6. Slice the wrap in half diagonally for easier handling.
7. Serve immediately or wrap tightly in parchment paper or aluminum foil for a portable lunch option.

- Customize the wrap with your favorite vegetables or spreads such as spinach, bell peppers, or salsa.
- Use leftover roasted turkey or chicken for a quick and convenient meal option.
- To prevent the wrap from getting soggy, layer the ingredients in the center of the tortilla and leave a border around the edges when spreading the hummus.

Nutritional Value (per serving):

- Calories: 300
- Protein: 20g
- Fat: 10g
- Carbohydrates: 30g
- Fiber: 6g
- Sugars: 4g

Health Benefits:

Lean Protein: Turkey breast is a lean source of protein, which helps build and repair tissues, support muscle growth, and keep you feeling full and satisfied.

Whole Grains: Whole wheat tortillas provide complex carbohydrates and dietary fiber, which contribute to sustained energy levels and promote digestive health.

Cooking Tips:

- Choose a whole wheat tortilla for added fiber and nutrients.

Vegetables: The wrap is packed with a variety of vegetables such as lettuce, cucumber, tomato, and red onion, providing essential vitamins, minerals, and antioxidants.

Heart-Healthy Fats: Hummus adds creamy texture and flavor to the wrap while providing heart-healthy fats from olive oil and tahini.

Portable and Convenient: This turkey and hummus wrap is perfect for on-the-go lunches, picnics, or packed lunches, providing a balanced and nutritious meal option that's easy to prepare and enjoy anywhere.

Enjoy this Turkey and Hummus Wrap with Whole Wheat Tortilla as a delicious and satisfying lunch option that's packed with flavor, protein, and wholesome ingredients.

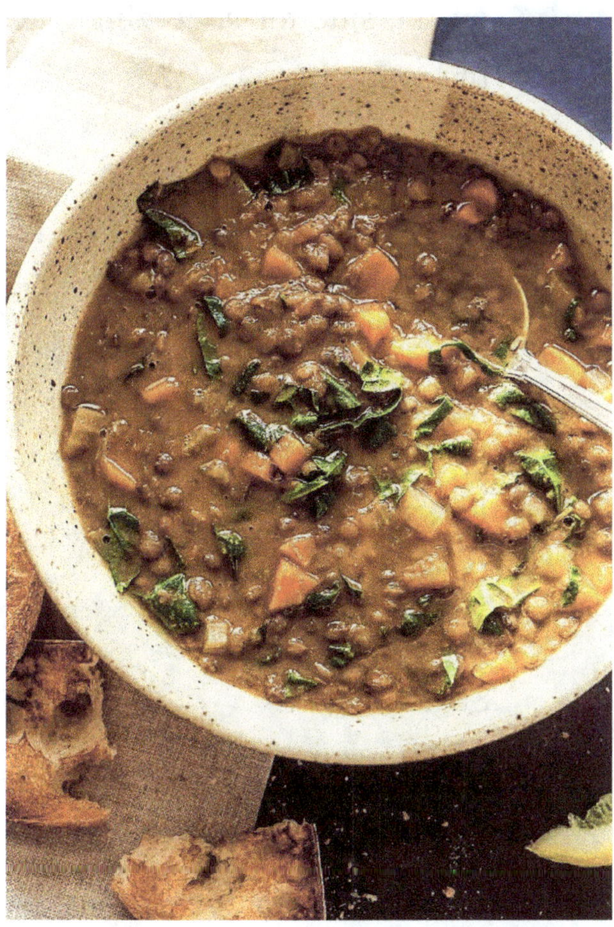

Time of Preparation: 10 minutes
Cooking Time: 30 minutes
Serving Unit: 4 servings

Ingredients:

- 1 cup dried green or brown lentils, rinsed and drained
- 1 tablespoon olive oil
- 1 onion, diced
- 2 cloves garlic, minced
- 2 carrots, diced
- 2 celery stalks, diced
- 1 teaspoon ground cumin
- 1/2 teaspoon ground coriander
- 1/2 teaspoon smoked paprika
- 1/4 teaspoon cayenne pepper (optional, for heat)
- 4 cups vegetable broth
- 1 can (14 oz) diced tomatoes
- 2 cups baby spinach or kale, chopped
- Salt and pepper to taste
- Fresh parsley for garnish (optional)
- Lemon wedges for serving (optional)

Procedure:

1. Heat olive oil in a large pot or Dutch oven over medium heat.
2. Add diced onion, garlic, carrots, and celery to the pot. Sauté until vegetables are softened, about 5-7 minutes.
3. Add ground cumin, ground coriander, smoked paprika, and cayenne pepper (if using) to the pot. Stir to coat the vegetables in the spices and cook for another 1-2 minutes until fragrant.
4. Add dried lentils, vegetable broth, and diced tomatoes to the pot. Bring to a boil, then reduce heat to low, cover, and simmer for 20-25 minutes or until lentils are tender.
5. Stir in chopped spinach or kale and cook for an additional 5 minutes until wilted.
6. Season the lentil soup with salt and pepper to taste.
7. Ladle the soup into bowls and garnish with fresh parsley if desired.
8. Serve hot with lemon wedges on the side for squeezing over the soup.

Nutritional Value (per serving):

- Calories: 250
- Protein: 15g
- Fat: 5g
- Carbohydrates: 40g
- Fiber: 15g
- Sugars: 8g

Cooking Tips:

1. Use green or brown lentils for this soup, as they hold their shape well when cooked and provide a hearty texture.
2. Customize the soup with your favorite vegetables such as bell peppers, zucchini, or potatoes.

3. Add extra broth or water if you prefer a thinner soup consistency.

4. For a creamier texture, blend a portion of the soup with an immersion blender or countertop blender before serving.

Health Benefits:

Plant-Based Protein: Lentils are a rich source of plant-based protein, which helps support muscle repair and growth.

High Fiber: Lentils are high in dietary fiber, which supports digestive health, regulates blood sugar levels, and promotes satiety.

Nutrient-Dense Vegetables: The soup is packed with nutrient-rich vegetables such as carrots, celery, spinach, and tomatoes, providing essential vitamins, minerals, and antioxidants.

Low in Fat: With minimal added fat, this lentil soup is relatively low in calories and fat, making it suitable for individuals watching their fat intake or looking to maintain a healthy weight.

Heart-Healthy: Lentils are cholesterol-free and low in saturated fat, making them a heart-healthy protein source that may help reduce the risk of cardiovascular disease.

Warm up with a comforting bowl of Lentil Soup with Vegetables, a wholesome and nutritious lunch option that's perfect for chilly days or anytime you crave a satisfying and nourishing meal.

Tuna Salad Lettuce Wraps

Ingredients:

- 1 can (5 oz) tuna in water, drained
- 2 tablespoons plain Greek yogurt
- 1 tablespoon mayonnaise (optional)
- 1 tablespoon Dijon mustard
- 1 celery stalk, finely chopped
- 1 tablespoon red onion, finely chopped
- 1 tablespoon fresh parsley, chopped
- Salt and pepper to taste
- 4 large lettuce leaves (such as romaine or butter lettuce)
- Optional toppings: sliced tomato, avocado, or cucumber

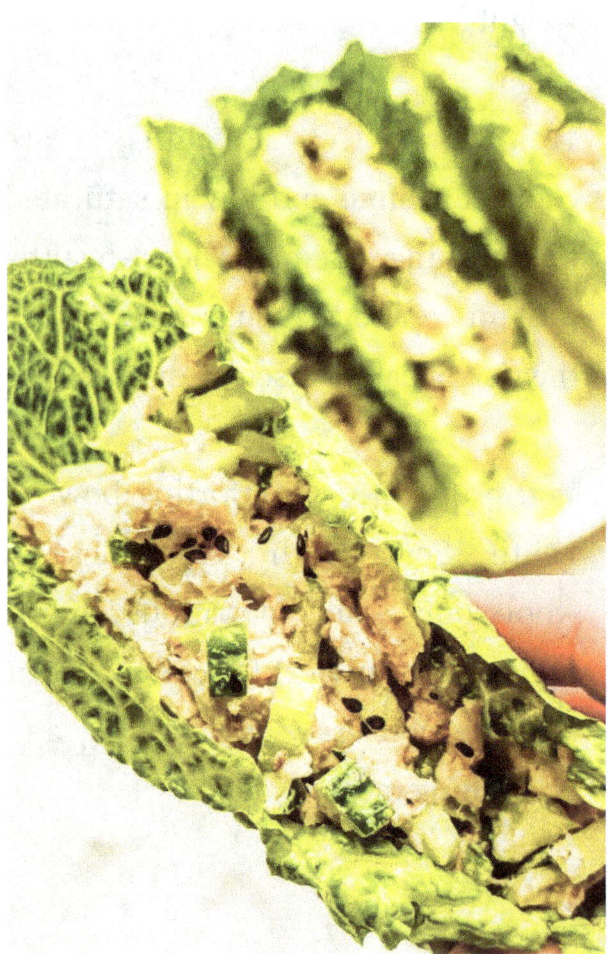

Time of Preparation: 15 minutes

Serving Unit: 2 lettuce wraps

Procedure:

1. In a mixing bowl, combine drained tuna, plain Greek yogurt, mayonnaise (if using), Dijon mustard, chopped celery,

chopped red onion, and chopped parsley. Mix until well combined.

2. Season the tuna salad with salt and pepper to taste.
3. Lay out the lettuce leaves on a clean work surface.
4. Divide the tuna salad mixture evenly among the lettuce leaves, spooning it onto the center of each leaf.
5. If desired, add sliced tomato, avocado, or cucumber on top of the tuna salad.
6. Roll up the lettuce leaves tightly, tucking in the sides as you go to enclose the filling.
7. Slice each lettuce wrap in half diagonally for easier handling.
8. Serve immediately or wrap tightly in parchment paper or aluminum foil for a portable lunch option.

Nutritional Value (per serving, One lettuce wrap):

- Calories: 150
- Protein: 15g
- Fat: 5g
- Carbohydrates: 8g
- Fiber: 2g
- Sugars: 2g

Cooking Tips:

1. Choose high-quality canned tuna packed in water for the best flavor and texture.
2. Greek yogurt adds creaminess and protein to the tuna salad without extra calories or fat. You can adjust the amount of mayonnaise or omit it entirely according to your preference.
3. Customize the tuna salad with your favorite mix-ins such as diced pickles, capers, or bell peppers.
4. For added flavor and crunch, sprinkle with a squeeze of fresh lemon juice or a dash of hot sauce before rolling up the lettuce wraps.

Health Benefits:

Protein-Rich: Tuna is a lean source of protein, which helps build and repair tissues, support muscle growth, and keep you feeling full and satisfied.

Low in Carbohydrates: Tuna salad lettuce wraps are naturally low in carbohydrates, making them suitable for individuals following a low-carb or ketogenic diet.

Healthy Fats: Tuna provides heart-healthy omega-3 fatty acids, which have been linked to reduced inflammation and improved heart health.

4. **High in Vitamins and Minerals:** Tuna is rich in essential nutrients such as vitamin D, vitamin B12, selenium, and iodine, which are important for overall health and well-being.

Light and Refreshing: Lettuce wraps provide a light and refreshing alternative to traditional sandwich bread or wraps, making them perfect for a lighter lunch option or for those looking to reduce their calorie intake.

Enjoy these Tuna Salad Lettuce Wraps as a light and satisfying lunch option that's perfect for a quick and healthy meal on busy days or anytime you crave a nutritious and delicious bite.

3

Dinner Entrees

Greetings, and welcome to "Chapter 3: Dinner Entrees," where we will be discussing a delightful assortment of main courses that are intended to take your evening meals to the next level. Beginning with hearty stews and progressing to succulent grilled dishes and flavorful pasta creations, this chapter is a culinary journey through a variety of dinner options that are both satisfying and wholesome.

Learn how to take pleasure in preparing meals that are not only nourishing but also delicious, and that bring both comfort and joy to your dinner table. Each recipe has been carefully crafted, incorporating fresh ingredients, vibrant flavors, and straightforward cooking techniques in order to assist you in creating unforgettable dining experiences for yourself and the people you care about.

Whether you are looking for ideas for a cozy dinner during the week or you are planning a special meal for guests, these dinner entrees offer something for every occasion and every palate. Come along with us as we are about to embark on a culinary journey that will be full of flavor, creativity, and the pleasure of sharing nourishing meals with the people you hold dear.

Baked Salmon with Lemon and Dill

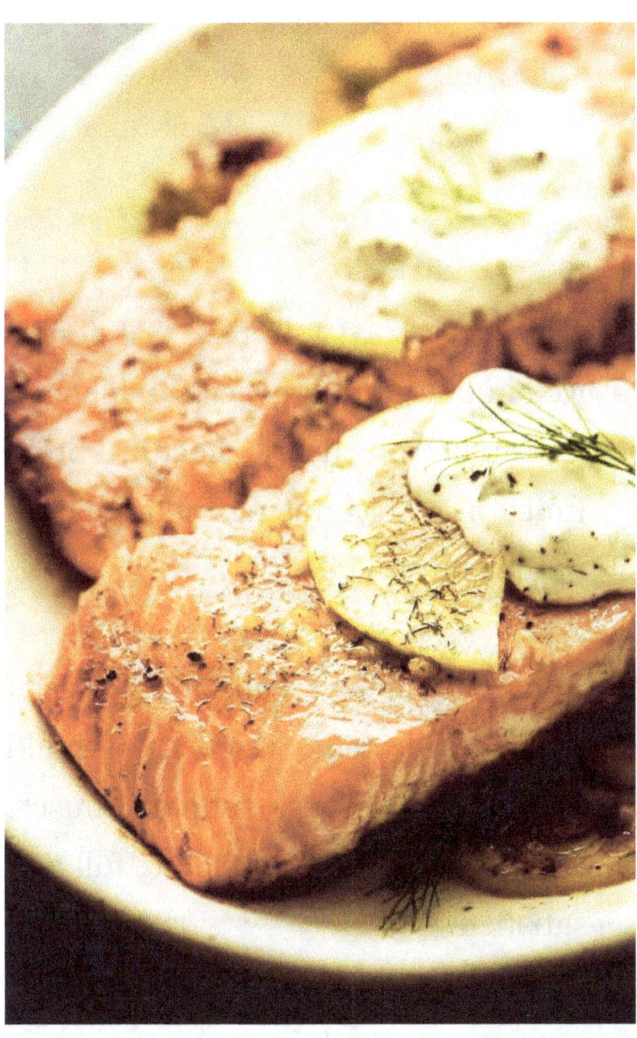

Time of Preparation: 10 minutes
Cooking Time: 15 minutes
Serving Unit: 2 servings

Ingredients:

- 2 salmon fillets (about 6 oz each), skin-on
- 1 tablespoon olive oil
- 1 lemon, thinly sliced
- tablespoons fresh dill, chopped
- Salt and pepper to taste

Procedure:

1. Preheat the oven to 400°F (200°C).
2. Place the salmon fillets on a baking sheet lined with parchment paper or aluminum foil.
3. Drizzle olive oil over the salmon fillets and season with salt and pepper to taste.
4. Arrange lemon slices on top of the salmon fillets and sprinkle with chopped fresh dill.
5. Bake in the preheated oven for 12-15 minutes or until the salmon is cooked through and flakes easily with a fork.

6. Remove from the oven and serve hot.

Nutritional Value (per serving):

- Calories: 300
- Protein: 30g
- Fat: 18g
- Carbohydrates: 2g
- Fiber: 1g
- Sugars: 0g

Cooking Tips:

1. Choose fresh, high-quality salmon fillets for the best flavor and texture.
2. Adjust the cooking time depending on the thickness of the salmon fillets. Thicker fillets may require additional cooking time.
3. Use fresh dill for optimal flavor, but dried dill can be used as a substitute if necessary.

4. Serve the baked salmon with a side of steamed vegetables or a mixed green salad for a balanced meal.

Health Benefits:

Omega-3 Fatty Acids: Salmon is rich in omega-3 fatty acids, which are essential for heart health, brain function, and reducing inflammation in the body.

Lean Protein: Salmon is a lean source of protein, which helps build and repair tissues, support muscle growth, and keep you feeling full and satisfied.

Vitamins and Minerals: Salmon is packed with essential nutrients such as vitamin D, vitamin B12, selenium, and potassium, which are important for overall health and well-being.

Low in Carbohydrates: This baked salmon recipe is naturally low in carbohydrates, making it suitable for individuals following a low-carb or ketogenic diet.

Quick and Easy: With just a few simple ingredients and minimal prep time, this baked salmon recipe is perfect for busy weeknights or special occasions when you want a delicious and nutritious meal without a lot of fuss.

Savor the flavors of this Baked Salmon with Lemon and Dill for a light and refreshing dinner option that's both elegant and easy to prepare.

Cauliflower Crust Pizza with Tomato and Basil

Time of Preparation: 20 minutes
Cooking Time: 25 minutes
Serving Unit: 2 servings (1 small pizza)

Ingredients:

1 small head cauliflower, riced (about 2 cups)
1 egg, lightly beaten
1/4 cup grated Parmesan cheese
1/2 teaspoon dried oregano
1/2 teaspoon garlic powder
Salt and pepper to taste
1/4 cup marinara sauce
1/2 cup shredded mozzarella cheese
1 roma tomato, thinly sliced
2-3 fresh basil leaves, torn

Procedure:

- Preheat the oven to 400°F (200°C). Line a baking sheet with parchment paper.
- In a large mixing bowl, combine the riced cauliflower, beaten egg, grated Parmesan cheese, dried oregano, garlic powder, salt, and pepper. Mix until well combined.
- Transfer the cauliflower mixture to the prepared baking sheet and spread it out evenly to form a circle, about 1/4 inch thick.
- Bake the cauliflower crust in the preheated oven for 20-25 minutes or until golden brown and firm.
- Remove the cauliflower crust from the oven and spread marinara sauce evenly over the surface.
- Sprinkle shredded mozzarella cheese over the marinara sauce.

- Arrange tomato slices on top of the cheese and sprinkle with torn fresh basil leaves.
- Return the pizza to the oven and bake for an additional 5-7 minutes or until the cheese is melted and bubbly.
- Remove from the oven, slice, and serve hot.

Nutritional Value (per serving):

- Calories: 200
- Protein: 15g
- Fat: 10g
- Carbohydrates: 15g
- Fiber: 5g
- Sugars: 5g

Cooking Tips:

1. Ensure the cauliflower crust is thoroughly cooked and golden brown before adding toppings to prevent it from becoming soggy.
2. Customize the pizza with your favorite toppings such as mushrooms, bell peppers, onions, or olives.
3. For a crispier crust, bake the cauliflower crust on a pizza stone or directly on the oven rack.
4. Use fresh basil leaves for a burst of flavor and aroma, but dried basil can be used as a substitute if necessary.

Health Benefits:

Low-Carb Alternative:
Cauliflower crust pizza is a low-carb alternative to traditional pizza crust, making it suitable for individuals following a low-carb or ketogenic diet.

Gluten-Free: Cauliflower crust pizza is naturally gluten-free, making it suitable for individuals with gluten intolerance or celiac disease.

High in Fiber: Cauliflower is rich in dietary fiber, which supports digestive health, regulates blood sugar levels, and promotes satiety.

Vitamins and Minerals:
Cauliflower is packed with essential nutrients such as vitamin C, vitamin K, folate, and potassium, which are important for overall health and well-being.

Vegetarian Option: Cauliflower crust pizza is a vegetarian-friendly option that provides protein from cheese and eggs while still delivering plenty of flavor and satisfaction.

Indulge in this Cauliflower Crust Pizza with Tomato and Basil for a delicious and guilt-free dinner option that's perfect for pizza lovers looking to enjoy a lighter and healthier alternative.

Time of Preparation: 20 minutes
Cooking Time: 20 minutes
Serving Unit: 4 servings

Ingredients:

For the Turkey Meatballs:

- 1 lb lean ground turkey
- 1/4 cup breadcrumbs (whole wheat or gluten-free)
- 1/4 cup grated Parmesan cheese
- 1 egg, lightly beaten
- 2 cloves garlic, minced
- 2 tablespoons fresh parsley, chopped
- 1 teaspoon dried oregano
- 1/2 teaspoon onion powder
- Salt and pepper to taste
- Olive oil for cooking

For the Zucchini Noodles:

- 4 medium zucchini
- 2 tablespoons olive oil
- 2 cloves garlic, minced
- Salt and pepper to taste

For Serving:

- Marinara sauce (store-bought or homemade)
- Fresh basil leaves for garnish
- Grated Parmesan cheese for topping

Procedure:

For the Turkey Meatballs:

1. Preheat the oven to 400°F (200°C). Line a baking sheet with parchment paper.
2. In a large mixing bowl, combine ground turkey, breadcrumbs, grated Parmesan cheese, beaten egg, minced garlic, chopped parsley, dried oregano, onion powder, salt,

and pepper. Mix until well combined.

3. Shape the turkey mixture into meatballs, about 1 inch in diameter, and place them on the prepared baking sheet.

4. Drizzle olive oil over the meatballs and bake in the preheated oven for 15-20 minutes or until cooked through and lightly browned.

For the Zucchini Noodles:

1. Trim the ends of the zucchini and spiralize them into noodles using a spiralizer.

2. Heat olive oil in a large skillet over medium heat. Add minced garlic and sauté for 1-2 minutes until fragrant.

3. Add the zucchini noodles to the skillet and toss to coat in the garlic-infused oil. Cook for 3-5 minutes until the noodles are tender but still slightly crisp. Season with salt and pepper to taste.

For Serving:

1. Serve the turkey meatballs over the zucchini noodles.

2. Spoon marinara sauce over the meatballs and noodles.

3. Garnish with fresh basil leaves and grated Parmesan cheese.

4. Serve hot and enjoy!

Nutritional Value (per serving):

- Calories: 300
- Protein: 25g
- Fat: 15g
- Carbohydrates: 15g
- Fiber: 3g
- Sugars: 5g

Cooking Tips:

1. Use lean ground turkey for healthier meatballs with less fat.

2. Feel free to customize the meatball seasoning with your favorite herbs and spices.

3. Make sure to thoroughly drain excess moisture from the zucchini noodles after spiralizing to prevent them from becoming watery when cooked.

4. For a quicker option, you can use store-bought zucchini noodles instead of spiralizing your own.

Health Benefits:

Lean Protein: Turkey meatballs are a lean source of protein, which helps build and repair tissues, support muscle growth, and keep you feeling full and satisfied.

Low-Carb Alternative: Zucchini noodles are a low-carb alternative to traditional pasta, making this dish suitable for individuals following a low-carb or ketogenic diet.

High in Fiber: Zucchini is rich in dietary fiber, which supports digestive health, regulates blood sugar levels, and promotes satiety.

Vitamins and Minerals: Zucchini is packed with essential nutrients such as vitamin C, vitamin K, potassium, and manganese, which are important for overall health and well-being.

Vegetable-Rich: This dish is packed with vegetables from the zucchini noodles and marinara sauce, providing essential vitamins, minerals, and antioxidants for optimal health.

Enjoy this flavorful and nutritious Turkey Meatballs with Zucchini Noodles for a satisfying dinner option that's both wholesome and delicious.

Stir-Fried Tofu with Broccoli and Bell Peppers

Time of Preparation: 15 minutes
Cooking Time: 15 minutes
Serving Unit: 2 servings

Ingredients:

- 1 block (14 oz) firm tofu, drained and pressed
- 2 tablespoons soy sauce (low-sodium if preferred)
- 1 tablespoon rice vinegar
- 1 tablespoon hoisin sauce
- 1 tablespoon sesame oil
- 2 cloves garlic, minced
- 1 teaspoon fresh ginger, grated
- 1 tablespoon cornstarch
- 2 tablespoons water
- 2 tablespoons vegetable oil
- 2 cups broccoli florets
- 1 bell pepper (any color), thinly sliced
- Cooked brown rice for serving
- Optional garnishes: sliced green onions, sesame seeds

Procedure:

- Cut the pressed tofu into cubes and place them on a clean kitchen towel or paper towels to absorb excess moisture.
- In a small bowl, whisk together soy sauce, rice vinegar, hoisin sauce, sesame oil, minced garlic, and grated ginger to make the sauce.
- In another small bowl, mix together cornstarch and water to make a slurry.
- Heat vegetable oil in a large skillet or wok over medium-high heat.
- Add the tofu cubes to the skillet and cook until golden brown and crispy on all sides, about 5-7 minutes. Remove tofu from the skillet and set aside.
- In the same skillet, add broccoli florets and sliced bell pepper.

Stir-fry for 3-4 minutes until vegetables are tender-crisp.

- Return the tofu to the skillet and pour the sauce over the tofu and vegetables.
- Stir in the cornstarch slurry and cook for another 2-3 minutes until the sauce has thickened and coats the tofu and vegetables evenly.
- Remove from heat and serve hot over cooked brown rice.
- Garnish with sliced green onions and sesame seeds if desired.

Nutritional Value (per serving):

- Calories: 300
- Protein: 15g
- Fat: 15g
- Carbohydrates: 25g
- Fiber: 5g
- Sugars: 5g

Cooking Tips:

Pressing tofu helps remove excess moisture and allows it to absorb more flavor during cooking.

Use firm tofu for stir-frying to prevent it from crumbling or falling apart.

Customize the stir-fry with your favorite vegetables such as carrots, snow peas, or mushrooms.

Serve the stir-fry over cooked brown rice for a complete and satisfying meal.

Health Benefits:

Plant-Based Protein: Tofu is a plant-based protein source, which provides essential amino acids necessary for building and repairing tissues.

Heart-Healthy Fats: Sesame oil adds rich flavor and heart-healthy fats to the stir-fry, which may help reduce the risk of heart disease.

Vegetable-Rich: This stir-fry is packed with vegetables like broccoli and bell peppers, providing essential vitamins, minerals, and antioxidants for optimal health.

Low-Calorie: Tofu and vegetables are low in calories but high in volume, making this stir-fry a filling and nutritious option for weight management.

Balanced Meal: Serving the stir-fry over brown rice adds complex carbohydrates and fiber, creating a balanced meal that provides sustained energy and satiety.

Enjoy the flavors and textures of this Stir-Fried Tofu with Broccoli and Bell Peppers for a satisfying and nutritious dinner option that's both delicious and wholesome.

Shrimp and Vegetable Stir-Fry with Brown Rice

Time of Preparation: 15 minutes
Cooking Time: 15 minutes
Serving Unit: 2 servings

Ingredients:

- 8 oz medium shrimp, peeled and deveined
- 2 tablespoons soy sauce (low-sodium if preferred)
- 1 tablespoon rice vinegar
- 1 tablespoon hoisin sauce
- 1 tablespoon sesame oil
- 2 cloves garlic, minced
- 1 teaspoon fresh ginger, grated
- 1 tablespoon cornstarch
- 2 tablespoons water
- 2 tablespoons vegetable oil
- 2 cups mixed vegetables (such as bell peppers, broccoli, carrots, and snap peas)
- Cooked brown rice for serving
- Optional garnishes: sliced green onions, sesame seeds

Procedure:

1. In a small bowl, whisk together soy sauce, rice vinegar, hoisin sauce, sesame oil, minced garlic, and grated ginger to make the sauce.
2. In another small bowl, mix together cornstarch and water to make a slurry.
3. Heat vegetable oil in a large skillet or wok over medium-high heat.
4. Add shrimp to the skillet and cook until pink and opaque, about 2-3 minutes per side. Remove shrimp from the skillet and set aside.
5. In the same skillet, add mixed vegetables and stir-fry for 3-4 minutes until tender-crisp.
6. Return the cooked shrimp to the skillet and pour the sauce over the shrimp and vegetables.

7. Stir in the cornstarch slurry and cook for another 2-3 minutes until the sauce has thickened and coats the shrimp and vegetables evenly.

8. Remove from heat and serve hot over cooked brown rice.

9. Garnish with sliced green onions and sesame seeds if desired.

Nutritional Value (per serving):

- Calories: 300
- Protein: 20g
- Fat: 10g
- Carbohydrates: 35g
- Fiber: 5g
- Sugars: 5g

Cooking Tips:

1. Use fresh or frozen shrimp for this recipe. Thaw frozen shrimp under cold running water before cooking.

2. Customize the stir-fry with your favorite vegetables or whatever you have on hand.

3. Serve the shrimp and vegetable stir-fry over cooked brown rice for a complete and balanced meal.

4. Adjust the seasoning and spice level of the sauce to suit your taste preferences.

Health Benefits:

Lean Protein: Shrimp is a lean source of protein, which helps build and repair tissues, support muscle growth, and keep you feeling full and satisfied.

Heart-Healthy Fats: Sesame oil adds rich flavor and heart-healthy fats to the stir-fry, which may help reduce the risk of heart disease.

Vegetable-Rich: This stir-fry is packed with colorful mixed vegetables, providing essential vitamins, minerals, and antioxidants for optimal health.

Low-Calorie: Shrimp and vegetables are low in calories but high in volume, making this stir-fry a filling and nutritious option for weight management.

Balanced Meal: Serving the stir-fry over brown rice adds complex carbohydrates and fiber, creating a balanced meal that provides sustained energy and satiety.

Enjoy the vibrant colors and flavors of this Shrimp and Vegetable Stir-Fry with Brown Rice for a nutritious and satisfying dinner option that's both delicious and wholesome.

4

Side Dishes and Snacks

We would like to take this opportunity to welcome you to "Chapter 4: Side Dishes and Snacks," in which we will discuss a wide range of delectable accompaniments and tasty bites that can be used to complement your meals or indulge your cravings in between meals. This chapter provides a variety of options to tantalize your taste buds and keep you fueled throughout the day. These options range from flavorful side dishes that elevate any main course to wholesome snacks that provide a boost of energy.

Find innovative ways to incorporate nutritious ingredients into your snacks and side dishes, such as making vibrant salads and hearty soups, as well as satisfying dips and spreads. Whether you are looking for a light and refreshing side dish to accompany your dinner or a satisfying snack to enjoy while you are on the go, this chapter will provide you with a lot of ideas to choose from.

Please come along with us as we venture on an adventure into the world of snacks and side dishes, where each bite is a delightful adventure in terms of flavor and texture. These recipes, which range from roasted vegetables that are crispy to hummus that is creamy and everything in between, are sure to become fixtures in your collection of culinary creations.

Roasted Brussels Sprouts with Balsamic Glaze

Time of Preparation: 10 minutes
Cooking Time: 25 minutes
Serving Unit: 4 servings

Ingredients:

- 1 lb Brussels sprouts, trimmed and halved
- 2 tablespoons olive oil
- Salt and pepper to taste
- 2 tablespoons balsamic glaze
- Optional: grated Parmesan cheese for serving

Procedure:

1. Preheat the oven to 400°F (200°C).
2. In a large mixing bowl, toss Brussels sprouts with olive oil, salt, and pepper until evenly coated.
3. Spread the Brussels sprouts in a single layer on a baking sheet lined with parchment paper.
4. Roast in the preheated oven for 20-25 minutes, tossing halfway through, until Brussels sprouts are tender and caramelized.
5. Remove from the oven and drizzle with balsamic glaze.
6. Serve hot, optionally garnished with grated Parmesan cheese.

Nutritional Value (per serving):

- Calories: 100
- Protein: 4g
- Fat: 6g
- Carbohydrates: 10g
- Fiber: 4g
- Sugars: 4g

Cooking Tips:

1. Trim the ends of the Brussels sprouts and remove any outer

leaves that are wilted or discolored.

2. Make sure to spread the Brussels sprouts in a single layer on the baking sheet to ensure even roasting.

3. Adjust the cooking time depending on the size of the Brussels sprouts and your desired level of caramelization.

4. For added flavor, sprinkle grated Parmesan cheese over the roasted Brussels sprouts before serving.

Health Benefits:

High in Fiber: Brussels sprouts are rich in dietary fiber, which supports digestive health, regulates blood sugar levels, and promotes satiety.

Vitamins and Minerals: Brussels sprouts are packed with essential nutrients such as vitamin C, vitamin K, folate, and potassium, which are important for overall health and well-being.

Antioxidants: Brussels sprouts contain antioxidants such as vitamin C and beta-carotene, which help protect cells from damage caused by free radicals and may reduce the risk of chronic diseases.

Low in Calories: Roasted Brussels sprouts are low in calories but high in volume, making them a filling and nutritious side dish option for weight management.

Heart-Healthy: Brussels sprouts are cholesterol-free and low in saturated fat, making them a heart-healthy addition to your diet that may help reduce the risk of cardiovascular disease.

Enjoy the caramelized sweetness of Roasted Brussels Sprouts with Balsamic Glaze as a flavorful and nutritious side dish that's perfect for any meal.

Cucumber and Tomato Salad with Feta Cheese

Time of Preparation: 10 minutes
Serving Unit: 4 servings

Ingredients:

- 2 large cucumbers, thinly sliced
- 2 cups cherry tomatoes, halved
- 1/4 cup red onion, thinly sliced
- 1/4 cup fresh parsley, chopped
- 1/4 cup crumbled feta cheese
- 2 tablespoons extra virgin olive oil
- 1 tablespoon red wine vinegar
- Salt and pepper to taste

Procedure:

- In a large mixing bowl, combine sliced cucumbers, halved cherry tomatoes, sliced red onion, and chopped parsley.
- In a small bowl, whisk together extra virgin olive oil, red wine vinegar, salt, and pepper to make the dressing.
- Pour the dressing over the cucumber and tomato mixture and toss until evenly coated.
- Sprinkle crumbled feta cheese over the salad and gently toss to combine.
- Serve chilled or at room temperature.

Nutritional Value (per serving):

- Calories: 100
- Protein: 3g
- Fat: 7g
- Carbohydrates: 8g
- Fiber: 2g
- Sugars: 4g

Cooking Tips:

1. Use fresh, ripe tomatoes and crisp cucumbers for the best flavor and texture.
2. Customize the salad with your favorite herbs and additional vegetables such as bell peppers, olives, or avocado.
3. For a creamier dressing, add a dollop of Greek yogurt or mayonnaise to the dressing mixture.
4. Allow the salad to marinate in the refrigerator for at least 30 minutes before serving to allow the flavors to meld together.

Health Benefits:

Hydration: Cucumbers and tomatoes have high water content, making this salad a hydrating option that helps maintain fluid balance and promotes healthy skin.

Vitamins and Minerals:
Cucumbers and tomatoes are rich in essential nutrients such as vitamin C, vitamin K, potassium, and antioxidants, which support overall health and well-being.

Low in Calories: This salad is low in calories but high in volume, making it a filling and nutritious option for weight management.

Heart-Healthy Fats: Olive oil provides heart-healthy monounsaturated fats, which may help reduce the risk of heart disease and inflammation in the body.

Bone Health: Feta cheese is a good source of calcium and phosphorus, which are important for bone health and strength.

Enjoy the crisp and refreshing flavors of Cucumber and Tomato Salad with Feta Cheese as a light and nutritious side dish that pairs perfectly with any meal.

Air-Fried Sweet Potato Fries

Time of Preparation: 10 minutes
Cooking Time: 15 minutes
Serving Unit: 4 servings

Ingredients:

- 2 large sweet potatoes, peeled and cut into fries
- 2 tablespoons olive oil
- 1 teaspoon paprika
- 1/2 teaspoon garlic powder
- 1/2 teaspoon onion powder
- Salt and pepper to taste
- Optional: chopped fresh parsley for garnish

Procedure:

1. In a large mixing bowl, toss sweet potato fries with olive oil, paprika, garlic powder, onion powder, salt, and pepper until evenly coated.
2. Preheat the air fryer to 400°F (200°C).
3. Place the seasoned sweet potato fries in the air fryer basket in a single layer, making sure not to overcrowd.
4. Cook in the preheated air fryer for 12-15 minutes, shaking the basket halfway through, until fries are crispy and golden brown.
5. Remove from the air fryer and transfer to a serving plate.
6. Garnish with chopped fresh parsley if desired.
7. Serve hot and enjoy!

Nutritional Value (per serving):

- Calories: 150
- Protein: 2g
- Fat: 7g
- Carbohydrates: 20g
- Fiber: 3g
- Sugars: 6g

Cooking Tips:

1. Cut the sweet potato fries into uniform sizes to ensure even cooking.
2. Season the fries generously with spices for maximum flavor.
3. Avoid overcrowding the air fryer basket to allow proper air circulation and ensure crispy fries.
4. Serve the sweet potato fries immediately after cooking for the best texture and flavor.

Health Benefits:

Rich in Vitamins: Sweet potatoes are rich in vitamins A and C, which are important for immune function, vision health, and skin health.

High in Fiber: Sweet potatoes are a good source of dietary fiber, which supports digestive health, regulates blood sugar levels, and promotes satiety.

Antioxidants: Sweet potatoes contain antioxidants such as beta-carotene and anthocyanins, which help protect cells from damage caused by free radicals and may reduce the risk of chronic diseases.

Heart-Healthy Fats: Olive oil provides heart-healthy monounsaturated fats, which may help reduce the risk of heart disease and inflammation in the body.

Gluten-Free: Sweet potato fries are naturally gluten-free, making them suitable for individuals with gluten intolerance or celiac disease.

Indulge in the crispy and flavorful goodness of Air-Fried Sweet Potato Fries as a healthier alternative to traditional french fries that's perfect for snacking or as a side dish.

Guacamole with Baked Tortilla Chips

Time of Preparation: 10 minutes

Cooking Time: 10 minutes

Serving Unit: 4 servings

Ingredients:

For the Guacamole:

- 2 ripe avocados, peeled and pitted
- 1 small tomato, diced
- 1/4 cup red onion, finely chopped
- 1/4 cup fresh cilantro, chopped
- 1 jalapeño pepper, seeded and minced (optional)
- 1 lime, juiced
- Salt and pepper to taste

For the Baked Tortilla Chips:

- 4 small corn tortillas
- 1 tablespoon olive oil
- Salt to taste

Procedure:

For the Guacamole:

1. In a medium mixing bowl, mash the ripe avocados with a fork until smooth but still slightly chunky.
2. Add diced tomato, chopped red onion, chopped cilantro, minced jalapeño pepper (if using), and lime juice to the mashed avocado.
3. Season with salt and pepper to taste and stir until well combined.
4. Cover the guacamole with plastic wrap, pressing it directly onto the surface to prevent browning.
5. Refrigerate for at least 30 minutes to allow the flavors to meld together.

For the Baked Tortilla Chips:

1. Preheat the oven to 375°F (190°C).
2. Brush both sides of each corn tortilla with olive oil and sprinkle with salt.
3. Stack the tortillas on top of each other and cut them into wedges using a sharp knife or pizza cutter.
4. Arrange the tortilla wedges in a single layer on a baking sheet lined with parchment paper.
5. Bake in the preheated oven for 8-10 minutes, flipping halfway through, until tortilla chips are crispy and golden brown.
6. Remove from the oven and let cool slightly before serving.

Nutritional Value (per serving, guacamole only):

- Calories: 150
- Protein: 2g
- Fat: 12g
- Carbohydrates: 10g
- Fiber: 7g
- Sugars: 2g

Cooking Tips:

1. Choose ripe avocados for the best flavor and texture. They should yield slightly to gentle pressure when squeezed.
2. Customize the guacamole with additional ingredients such as diced bell peppers, minced garlic, or chopped jalapeños for extra heat.
3. Serve the guacamole with baked tortilla chips or fresh vegetable crudites for dipping.
4. To prevent browning, store leftover guacamole in an airtight container with plastic wrap pressed directly onto the surface and refrigerate promptly.

Health Benefits:

Healthy Fats: Avocados are rich in heart-healthy monounsaturated fats, which help reduce inflammation and may lower the risk of heart disease.

Vitamins and Minerals: Avocados are packed with essential nutrients such as vitamin K, vitamin E, potassium, and folate, which support overall health and well-being.

Antioxidants: Tomatoes and onions contain antioxidants such as lycopene and quercetin, which help protect cells from damage caused by free radicals and may reduce the risk of chronic diseases.

Fiber-Rich: Guacamole is a good source of dietary fiber, which supports digestive health, regulates blood sugar levels, and promotes satiety.

Gluten-Free: Both guacamole and baked tortilla chips are naturally gluten-free, making them suitable for individuals with gluten intolerance or celiac disease.

Enjoy the creamy and flavorful goodness of Guacamole with Baked Tortilla Chips as a delicious and nutritious snack or appetizer that's perfect for sharing with friends and family.

5

Desserts and Treats

Presenting "Chapter 5: Desserts and Treats," where we'll savor life's sweeter side with a variety of delicious desserts and treats that will fulfill your sweet tooth without jeopardizing your health objectives. This chapter offers a range of choices to satisfy your sweet tooth and nourish your body, from rich desserts to guilt-free treats.

Learn how to make desserts that are lower in sugar, fat, and calories without compromising on flavor or satisfaction by following these delectable recipes that make use of healthy ingredients and clever substitutions. This chapter has plenty of inspiration, whether you're in the mood for a refreshing treat to cool off on a hot day or a classic dessert with a healthier twist.

Come along as we delve into the world of sweets and treats, where each morsel is a joyous celebration of flavor and texture. These recipes, which range from light and refreshing treats to rich and creamy desserts, are sure to become favorites for any occasion.

Sugar-Free Apple Crisp

Time of Preparation: 15 minutes
Cooking Time: 45 minutes
Serving Unit: 6 servings

Ingredients:

For the Apple Filling:

- 4 large apples, peeled, cored, and thinly sliced
- 2 tablespoons lemon juice
- 1 teaspoon ground cinnamon
- 1/4 teaspoon ground nutmeg
- 1 tablespoon cornstarch

For the Crisp Topping:

- 1 cup old-fashioned rolled oats
- 1/2 cup almond flour
- 1/4 cup chopped almonds
- 1/4 cup unsweetened shredded coconut
- 1/4 cup melted coconut oil
- 2 tablespoons maple syrup or sugar-free sweetener of choice
- 1 teaspoon ground cinnamon
- Pinch of salt

Procedure:

- Preheat the oven to 350°F (175°C). Grease a 9x9-inch baking dish with coconut oil or non-stick cooking spray.
- In a large mixing bowl, combine sliced apples, lemon juice, ground cinnamon, ground nutmeg, and cornstarch. Toss until the apples are evenly coated.
- Transfer the apple mixture to the prepared baking dish and spread it out into an even layer.
- In a separate mixing bowl, combine rolled oats, almond flour, chopped almonds, shredded coconut, melted coconut oil, maple syrup or sugar-free sweetener, ground

cinnamon, and salt. Mix until well combined and crumbly.

- Sprinkle the crisp topping evenly over the apple mixture in the baking dish.
- Bake in the preheated oven for 40-45 minutes, or until the topping is golden brown and the apples are tender.
- Remove from the oven and let cool slightly before serving.
- Serve warm, optionally topped with a dollop of Greek yogurt or a scoop of sugar-free vanilla ice cream.

Nutritional Value (per serving):

- Calories: 250
- Protein: 4g
- Fat: 14g
- Carbohydrates: 30g
- Fiber: 6g
- Sugars: 12g

Cooking Tips:

- Choose a mix of sweet and tart apples such as Honeycrisp, Granny Smith, or Fuji for the best flavor balance in the apple filling.
- Adjust the sweetness of the crisp topping to your preference by adding more or less maple syrup or sugar-free sweetener.
- Serve the apple crisp warm for the best texture and flavor, optionally topped with a scoop of your favorite sugar-free ice cream or whipped cream.
- Leftover apple crisp can be stored in an airtight container in the refrigerator for up to 3 days. Reheat before serving for the best taste and texture.

Health Benefits:

High in Fiber: Apples are rich in dietary fiber, which supports digestive health, regulates blood sugar levels, and promotes satiety.

Vitamins and Minerals: Apples are packed with essential nutrients such as vitamin C, vitamin K, potassium, and antioxidants, which are important for overall health and well-being.

Heart-Healthy Fats: Almonds and coconut oil provide heart-healthy monounsaturated fats and medium-chain triglycerides (MCTs), which may help reduce the risk of heart disease and improve cholesterol levels.

Low-Glycemic: This sugar-free apple crisp is sweetened with natural ingredients such as apples and maple syrup, making it a lower-glycemic option compared to traditional desserts sweetened with refined sugar.

Gluten-Free and Dairy-Free: This recipe is naturally gluten-free and dairy-free, making it suitable for individuals with gluten intolerance or lactose intolerance.

Indulge in the comforting flavors of Sugar-Free Apple Crisp as a guilt-free dessert option that's perfect for any occasion, from cozy nights in to special gatherings with loved ones.

Dark Chocolate Covered Strawberries

Time of Preparation: 15 minutes
Cooking Time: 5 minutes
Serving Unit: 12 strawberries

Ingredients:

- 12 large strawberries, rinsed and dried
- 4 oz dark chocolate, chopped (at least 70% cocoa)
- 1 teaspoon coconut oil
- Optional toppings: chopped nuts, shredded coconut, sea salt

Procedure:

1. Line a baking sheet with parchment paper.
2. In a heatproof bowl, combine chopped dark chocolate and coconut oil.
3. Microwave in 30-second intervals, stirring between each interval, until the chocolate is melted and smooth.
4. Holding each strawberry by the stem, dip it into the melted chocolate, coating about three-quarters of the berry.
5. Allow any excess chocolate to drip off, then place the dipped strawberry on the prepared baking sheet.
6. Repeat with the remaining strawberries.
7. If desired, sprinkle the dipped strawberries with chopped nuts, shredded coconut, or a pinch of sea salt while the chocolate is still wet.
8. Place the baking sheet in the refrigerator for about 15 minutes, or until the chocolate is set.
9. Once set, transfer the chocolate-covered strawberries to a serving plate.

10. Serve immediately, or store in the refrigerator until ready to serve.

Nutritional Value (per serving, Two strawberries):

- Calories: 120
- Protein: 1g
- Fat: 8g
- Carbohydrates: 12g
- Fiber: 3g
- Sugars: 8g

Cooking Tips:

1. Choose ripe strawberries that are firm and free from blemishes for the best results.
2. Use high-quality dark chocolate with at least 70% cocoa content for a rich and indulgent flavor.
3. Adding coconut oil to the melted chocolate helps create a smoother and shinier coating on the strawberries.
4. Customize the chocolate-covered strawberries with your favorite toppings, such as chopped nuts, shredded coconut, or a sprinkle of sea salt, for added flavor and texture.

Health Benefits:

Antioxidants: Dark chocolate is rich in antioxidants, such as flavonoids and polyphenols, which help protect cells from damage caused by free radicals and may reduce the risk of chronic diseases.

Heart Health: Consuming dark chocolate in moderation has been associated with improved heart health, including lower blood pressure and reduced risk of heart disease.

Vitamins and Minerals:

Strawberries are packed with essential nutrients such as vitamin C, manganese, and antioxidants, which support overall health and well-being.

Lower in Sugar: Compared to other desserts, dark chocolate-covered strawberries are relatively low in sugar, making them a healthier option for satisfying your sweet cravings.

Portion Control: Enjoying two or three chocolate-covered strawberries provides a satisfying sweet treat without overindulging in excess calories or sugar.

Savor the irresistible combination of juicy strawberries and rich dark chocolate with these Dark Chocolate Covered Strawberries, perfect for a romantic dessert or a sweet indulgence any time of the year.

Chia Seed Pudding with Berries

Time of Preparation: 5 minutes (plus chilling time)

Serving Unit: 2 servings

Ingredients:

- 1/4 cup chia seeds
- 1 cup unsweetened almond milk or coconut milk
- 1 tablespoon maple syrup or honey (optional)
- 1/2 teaspoon vanilla extract
- Fresh berries for topping (such as strawberries, blueberries, raspberries)

Procedure:

1. In a mixing bowl or glass jar, combine chia seeds, almond milk or coconut milk, maple syrup or honey (if using), and vanilla extract.
2. Stir well to combine, making sure the chia seeds are evenly distributed.
3. Cover the bowl or jar and refrigerate for at least 2 hours or overnight, allowing the chia seeds to absorb the liquid and thicken into a pudding-like consistency.
4. Stir the chia seed pudding before serving to redistribute the seeds.
5. Divide the chia seed pudding into serving bowls or glasses.
6. Top with fresh berries just before serving.

Nutritional Value (per serving):

- Calories: 150
- Protein: 4g
- Fat: 8g
- Carbohydrates: 15g
- Fiber: 10g
- Sugars: 4g

Cooking Tips:

1. Customize the chia seed pudding with your favorite sweeteners and flavorings, such as maple syrup, honey, vanilla extract, or cocoa powder.
2. Experiment with different types of milk alternatives, such as almond milk, coconut milk, or oat milk, to suit your dietary preferences.
3. For added flavor and texture, mix in toppings such as chopped nuts, shredded coconut, or sliced bananas before serving.
4. Prepare a batch of chia seed pudding in advance and store it in individual serving jars or containers for a quick and convenient breakfast or snack option.

Health Benefits:

Omega-3 Fatty Acids: Chia seeds are a rich source of omega-3 fatty acids, which are important for brain health, heart health, and reducing inflammation in the body.

Fiber-Rich: Chia seeds are high in dietary fiber, which supports digestive health, regulates blood sugar levels, and promotes satiety.

Protein: Chia seeds are a complete protein source, providing all nine essential amino acids necessary for building and repairing tissues.

Antioxidants: Berries such as strawberries, blueberries, and raspberries are rich in antioxidants, which help protect cells from damage caused by free radicals and may reduce the risk of chronic diseases.

Low-Glycemic: Chia seed pudding is naturally low in sugar and has a low glycemic index, making it a suitable option for individuals with diabetes or those watching their blood sugar levels.

Enjoy the creamy texture and refreshing taste of Chia Seed Pudding with Berries as a nutritious and satisfying dessert or snack that's both delicious and good for you.

30-Day Meal Plan

Week 1

Day 1

Breakfast: Veggie Omelette with Spinach and Mushrooms
Lunch: Grilled Chicken Salad with Balsamic Vinaigrette
Dinner: Baked Salmon with Lemon and Dill
Snack: Greek Yogurt and Fruit Smoothie

Day 2

Breakfast: Overnight Oats with Chia Seeds and Almond Milk
Lunch: Quinoa and Black Bean Stuffed Bell Peppers
Dinner: Cauliflower Crust Pizza with Tomato and Basil
Snack: Dark Chocolate Covered Strawberries

Day 3

Breakfast: Whole Wheat Pancakes with Sugar-Free Syrup
Lunch: Turkey and Hummus Wrap with Whole Wheat Tortilla
Dinner: Turkey Meatballs with Zucchini Noodles
Snack: Cucumber and Tomato Salad with Feta Cheese

Day 4

Breakfast: Avocado Toast with Poached Egg
Lunch: Lentil Soup with Vegetables
Dinner: Stir-Fried Tofu with Broccoli and Bell Peppers
Snack: Air-Fried Sweet Potato Fries

Day 5

Breakfast: Berry and Greek Yogurt Parfait
Lunch: Tuna Salad Lettuce Wraps
Dinner: Shrimp and Vegetable Stir-Fry with Brown Rice
Snack: Sugar-Free Apple Crisp

Day 6

Breakfast: Veggie Omelette with Spinach and Mushrooms
Lunch: Grilled Chicken Salad with Balsamic Vinaigrette
Dinner: Baked Salmon with Lemon and Dill
Snack: Guacamole with Baked Tortilla Chips

Day 7

Breakfast: Overnight Oats with Chia Seeds and Almond Milk
Lunch: Quinoa and Black Bean Stuffed Bell Peppers
Dinner: Cauliflower Crust Pizza with Tomato and Basil
Snack: Greek Yogurt Popsicles with Mango Puree

Day 8

Breakfast: Whole Wheat Pancakes with Sugar-Free Syrup
Lunch: Turkey and Hummus Wrap with Whole Wheat Tortilla
Dinner: Turkey Meatballs with Zucchini Noodles
Snack: Dark Chocolate Covered Strawberries

Day 9

Breakfast: Avocado Toast with Poached Egg
Lunch: Lentil Soup with Vegetables
Dinner: Stir-Fried Tofu with Broccoli and Bell Peppers
Snack: Cucumber and Tomato Salad with Feta Cheese

Breakfast: Berry and Greek Yogurt Parfait
Lunch: Tuna Salad Lettuce Wraps
Dinner: Shrimp and Vegetable Stir-Fry with Brown Rice
Snack: Air-Fried Sweet Potato Fries

Breakfast: Veggie Omelette with Spinach and Mushrooms
Lunch: Grilled Chicken Salad with Balsamic Vinaigrette
Dinner: Baked Salmon with Lemon and Dill
Snack: Sugar-Free Apple Crisp

Breakfast: Overnight Oats with Chia Seeds and Almond Milk
Lunch: Quinoa and Black Bean Stuffed Bell Peppers
Dinner: Cauliflower Crust Pizza with Tomato and Basil
Snack: Greek Yogurt Popsicles with Mango Puree

Breakfast: Whole Wheat Pancakes with Sugar-Free Syrup
Lunch: Turkey and Hummus Wrap with Whole Wheat Tortilla
Dinner: Turkey Meatballs with Zucchini Noodles
Snack: Dark Chocolate Covered Strawberries

Breakfast: Avocado Toast with Poached Egg
Lunch: Lentil Soup with Vegetables
Dinner: Stir-Fried Tofu with Broccoli and Bell Peppers
Snack: Guacamole with Baked Tortilla Chips

Week 3

Day 15

Breakfast: Berry and Greek Yogurt Parfait
Lunch: Tuna Salad Lettuce Wraps
Dinner: Shrimp and Vegetable Stir-Fry with Brown Rice
Snack: Air-Fried Sweet Potato Fries

Day 16

Breakfast: Veggie Omelette with Spinach and Mushrooms
Lunch: Grilled Chicken Salad with Balsamic Vinaigrette
Dinner: Baked Salmon with Lemon and Dill
Snack: Cucumber and Tomato Salad with Feta Cheese

Day 17

Breakfast: Overnight Oats with Chia Seeds and Almond Milk
Lunch: Quinoa and Black Bean Stuffed Bell Peppers
Dinner: Cauliflower Crust Pizza with Tomato and Basil
Snack: Greek Yogurt Popsicles with Mango Puree

Day 18

Breakfast: Whole Wheat Pancakes with Sugar-Free Syrup
Lunch: Turkey and Hummus Wrap with Whole Wheat Tortilla
Dinner: Turkey Meatballs with Zucchini Noodles
Snack: Dark Chocolate Covered Strawberries

Day 19

Breakfast: Avocado Toast with Poached Egg
Lunch: Lentil Soup with Vegetables
Dinner: Stir-Fried Tofu with Broccoli and Bell Peppers
Snack: Sugar-Free Apple Crisp

Day 20

Breakfast: Berry and Greek Yogurt Parfait
Lunch: Tuna Salad Lettuce Wraps
Dinner: Shrimp and Vegetable Stir-Fry with Brown Rice
Snack: Air-Fried Sweet Potato Fries

Day 21

Breakfast: Veggie Omelette with Spinach and Mushrooms
Lunch: Grilled Chicken Salad with Balsamic Vinaigrette
Dinner: Baked Salmon with Lemon and Dill
Snack: Guacamole with Baked Tortilla Chips

Day 22

Breakfast: Overnight Oats with Chia Seeds and Almond Milk
Lunch: Quinoa and Black Bean Stuffed Bell Peppers
Dinner: Cauliflower Crust Pizza with Tomato and Basil
Snack: Greek Yogurt Popsicles with Mango Puree

Day 23

Breakfast: Whole Wheat Pancakes with Sugar-Free Syrup
Lunch: Turkey and Hummus Wrap with Whole Wheat Tortilla
Dinner: Turkey Meatballs with Zucchini Noodles
Snack: Dark Chocolate Covered Strawberries

Day 24

Breakfast: Avocado Toast with Poached Egg
Lunch: Lentil Soup with Vegetables
Dinner: Stir-Fried Tofu with Broccoli and Bell Peppers
Snack: Cucumber and Tomato Salad with Feta Cheese

Day 25

Breakfast: Berry and Greek Yogurt Parfait
Lunch: Tuna Salad Lettuce Wraps
Dinner: Shrimp and Vegetable Stir-Fry with Brown Rice
Snack: Air-Fried Sweet Potato Fries

Day 26

Breakfast: Veggie Omelette with Spinach and Mushrooms
Lunch: Grilled Chicken Salad with Balsamic Vinaigrette
Dinner: Baked Salmon with Lemon and Dill
Snack: Sugar-Free Apple Crisp

Day 27

Breakfast: Overnight Oats with Chia Seeds and Almond Milk
Lunch: Quinoa and Black Bean Stuffed Bell Peppers
Dinner: Cauliflower Crust Pizza with Tomato and Basil
Snack: Greek Yogurt Popsicles with Mango Puree

Day 28

Breakfast: Whole Wheat Pancakes with Sugar-Free Syrup
Lunch: Turkey and Hummus Wrap with Whole Wheat Tortilla
Dinner: Turkey Meatballs with Zucchini Noodles
Snack: Dark Chocolate Covered Strawberries

Day 29

Breakfast: Avocado Toast with Poached Egg
Lunch: Lentil Soup with Vegetables
Dinner: Stir-Fried Tofu with Broccoli and Bell Peppers

Snack: Guacamole with Baked
Tortilla Chips

Day 30

Breakfast: Berry and Greek Yogurt
Parfait
Lunch: Tuna Salad Lettuce Wraps
Dinner: Shrimp and Vegetable Stir-
Fry with Brown Rice
Snack: Air-Fried Sweet Potato Fries

Conclusion

As we reach the end of our journey through the world of "Simple and Easy Diabetic Diet After 50," it's important to reflect on the valuable lessons learned and the delicious recipes shared. This cookbook has been crafted with the intention of providing practical guidance and flavorful solutions for individuals managing diabetes or simply seeking healthier dietary choices, especially as they navigate life after 50.

Throughout these pages, we've explored a diverse array of recipes that prioritize simplicity, ease of preparation, and, above all, nutritional balance. From hearty breakfast ideas to satisfying dinner entrees, refreshing side dishes, and indulgent desserts, each recipe has been carefully curated to offer both nourishment and enjoyment.

One of the key themes woven into the fabric of this cookbook is the emphasis on whole, unprocessed ingredients. By incorporating plenty of fruits, vegetables, whole grains, lean proteins, and healthy fats into our meals, we not only support our overall health but also manage blood sugar levels more effectively.

Moreover, we've embraced the concept of moderation, recognizing that enjoying our favorite foods in reasonable portions can coexist harmoniously with a diabetic-friendly lifestyle. By making mindful choices and being mindful of portion sizes, we empower ourselves to savor the flavors we love without compromising our health goals.

As we bid farewell to these pages, let us carry forward the knowledge, inspiration, and culinary creativity gained from our exploration of "Simple and Easy Diabetic Diet After 50." Let us continue to nourish our bodies with wholesome foods, delight our taste buds with vibrant flavors, and celebrate the joy of eating well.

Remember, the journey to better health is not about deprivation or sacrifice but rather about making informed choices that nourish both body and soul. May this cookbook serve as a trusted companion on your path to wellness, offering guidance, inspiration, and, above all, the promise of delicious meals shared with loved ones.

Here's to good health, happy cooking, and a future filled with flavor!

Bon appétit!